It's Your Health

Navigating American Health Care

Robert D'Antonio Ph.D.

ISBN: 1453878165
ISBN-13: 9781453878163
Printed in the United States of America

Acknowledgements

This book is a direct result of the constant prodding by my friends to share my experiences in the health care industry. My desire to take charge of my life and to encourage others to take charge of and take responsibility for their health care comes from my parents. They taught me to be independent and responsible for my actions. Thanks Mom and Dad.

I thank Annette for including me in her life during a very difficult time, and Jack for his constant encouragement.

To Val Jean, who always has an intense desire to know and no fear of asking questions. She is never satisfied with mediocrity or indifference. She always has a plan and is dedicated to her family. Thanks, Val Jean.

I thank my two brothers, both physicians, who care for and about their patients.

My daughter, Natalie, whose kindness, generosity, and compassion serve as a constant reminder to me of how we should treat each other. Thanks, Hoodle.

Finally, my wife, Claire, who believes in me. She has always supported me. She is responsible for this book being published. Thank you, Claire. Love you.

Table of Contents

Chapter 1:
Health Care in the USA

What was that advertisement for Buick? This is not your father's Buick. This applies to health care in America. It is not your father's health care. Times have changed and in a very big way. Health care has become more complicated and more expensive. The industry has amazing diagnostic radiology machines, wonder drugs, new therapies, and amazing surgical techniques. Because of these incredible new treatments and technologies, patient survival has increased significantly. These new tools for the diagnostician and care provider come at a high price. Health care is more expensive than ever—more than your father could ever imagine.

Medicine has become highly specialized. All physicians receive basic medical training in medical school and during internship at a teaching institution. After their internships, physicians make a decision that directs their training and ultimately their lifelong practice to a very specific specialty. These men and women are intensely trained in one aspect of medical care like cardiology, for instance. The physician who chooses cardiology has a comprehensive residency and postdoctoral fellowship in the diagnosis and treatment of conditions and diseases of the human heart. Over the last forty years, this type of specific training has evolved to the point where patients in America can expect a cardiologist to be well trained and competent to treat any and all heart ailments. The result of this new approach to health care has increased the quality and effectiveness of medical care provided to the average American.

New surgical techniques are being developed every day. These digital (computer-aided) techniques are not as invasive as techniques used in the past. Tiny incisions are made and small cameras are inserted that are used to guide the surgeon's hand (arthroscopy or laparoscopy). Because of telemedicine, it is now possible to perform and/or assist in surgeries using the digital net between cities or even continents. Certain brain tumors are excised by a new technique called the gamma blade. The digital age is real and in widespread use in medicine.

During the last twenty-five years, the field of diagnostic radiology has exploded with new and remarkable machines. Computed automated tomography (CT scan), magnetic resonance imaging (MRI), nuclear imaging, positron emission tomography (PET), and the combination of CT and PET have given the radiologist an unbelievable ability to peer into the human body and identify abnormalities or diseases. Digital mammography has enabled physicians to diagnose breast cancer at a very early stage that equates to a higher survival rate for the stricken patient.

Pharmaceutical intervention has become a routine procedure for the treatment regime of many diseases.

There are drugs for just about every organ, bone, muscle, tendon, or physiological process, and they are being used extensively in the care of Americans today. The treatments for cardiovascular disorders and cancer have been greatly enhanced because of these wonder drugs, and it appears that more are on the horizon.

Radiation therapy, kidney dialysis, and organ transplants have given a terminally ill patient an extension on his or her longevity or in some diseases a normal life span.

All of these new medical procedures, diagnostic imaging modalities, and therapies have greatly increased the rate of survival and quality of life. But—and there is always a *but*—it is very expensive. For example, a new CT or MRI machine is over $1.75 million and a PET/CT machine is at least $2 million. The cost of developing a new drug is in the hundreds of millions of dollars. The men and women who have dedicated their lives to delivering care to Americans are highly trained. The cost of their education and training has also significantly increased over the last forty years. Thus, based on their training and responsibilities, their wages must reflect these aspects. The insurance companies that provide health insurance are publicly owned (traded on Wall Street) corporations and are designed to make a profit. Obviously, these new medical procedures, imaging modalities, wonder drugs, and therapies are incredibly expensive, and therefore the health insurance companies have established rules and guidelines to limit their exposure.

Okay, health care is now more effective but much more expensive. So, how do you navigate through the health care industry and survive? Good question. I believe you can do it by being well informed and vigilant about your health and those delivering your care, and knowing your rights as a patient.

Chapter 2:
Choosing Your Physician

The single most important aspect of your health care is ensuring that the right physician is caring for you. The decision process starts with you. You must determine what you need in a physician. Let me suggest a few questions to help you pick a physician.

Is the physician well trained?

There are only a few ways available to a patient to determine whether a physician is well trained. Obviously, the physician must be licensed to practice medicine in your state. A phone call or an e-mail to your state Medical Licensing Board will resolve this question quickly (see the list of state boards in appendix A).

Where did the physician train?

If he or she trained outside the United States, I recommend that you determine where the training occurred and if it is a reputable institution. If the training occurred within the United States, the physician should have certificates or diplomas from the institutions. If you cannot determine this issue for yourself, ask the physician. If the answer is vague or no to training, then I suggest that you seek another physician. The

American Medical Association (AMA) has a free service available on the Internet for information about physicians called AMA Physician Select (see appendix A).

Is my physician board certified?

Assuming the training issue is acceptable, then determine if the physician is board certified. To be board certified, the physician must pass a comprehensive test offered by the governing body of a specific specialty. The AMA, all the state health agencies, and the federal government recognize this body.

Board certification is a touchy issue within the medical community. Many older physicians feel that board certification is not indicative of a physician's abilities. They feel that there are many excellent physicians who are not board certified. I am sure that this is true. However, the public has so few mechanisms to determine whether a physician is competent, it would be logical for a patient to use board certification as a measure of a physician's ability. Each and every physician decides whether to sit for the board examination in his or her specialty. It is a personal decision that has nothing to do with the patient or patient care.

Because there are so few ways for a patient to determine the competency of a physician, I recommend that board certification be used. I see board certification as a demonstration of the physician's knowledge in his or her specialty and confidence in his or her abilities. You can find more information by visiting the Web site of the American Board of Medical Specialties (see appendix A or call 800-776-2378).

So now you have found a physician who is licensed in your state and is board certified. These next issues are the hardest. You must ask yourself "How do I want to be treated by the physician?" Do you want someone to hold your hand all the time or do you want someone who gives your diagnosis straight to you? I recommend that you find yourself a physician in the latter category who is also compassionate.

Look for a physician with the following qualities:

Gender: Same sex as you (although this is a highly debatable issue).

Age: Many people are most comfortable with doctors a little older than they are, although there are also many excellent young physicians; choose one with whom you feel comfortable.

Communication: A physician must be willing to explain your situation in terms that you understand and must be patient enough to explain the issues repeatedly until you do understand. Your appointment with the physician should not have a time limit but be exactly as long as it takes for you and the physician to be satisfied that good communication occurred between the two of you. He or she should be able to give you information concerning your health in such a way as to be considerate of your fears and feelings while ensuring that all the facts are included: heavy sugar coating will not help you in the long run. He or she must give you his or her opinion as to the course of treatment you should take.

The physician should be willing to speak to you on the telephone. You should expect your primary care physician to be your advocate with other care providers, hospitals, and insurance companies.

Physician's Staff: Most importantly, the physician's staff must reflect all of the traits of the physician—good communication, educator, compassion/caring, and your advocate.

Reputation: Finally, you should speak to friends and family about the physician. It is very likely that if your friends or family are like you, and they feel strongly about a physician, you will also feel the same way.

Get Acquainted Appointment: Once you have chosen a new primary care physician, you should call and make an appointment to meet him or her and determine whether the two of you will be compatible.

Any physician's office that refuses to make this type of appointment should be avoided. The relationship between a physician and a patient must be based on trust. If you cannot get one short meeting with the physician to determine this compatibility issue, then I suggest that you will never have the relationship that is needed to secure good health care.

I recommend that every person have a primary care physician. Usually, this is an internal medicine or family practice specialist. Regardless of which type of physician you choose, the individual should be board certified. This physician should be willing to be your gatekeeper.

At least once a year, you should see your primary care physician and receive a full physical examination. He or she is the only physician trained to take all of the pieces of medical information and formulate/control a plan of care. Upon his or her diagnosis, the primary care physician will refer you to the appropriate specialist.

It is essential that your primary care physician receive all the medical information from the specialist; unfortunately, not all specialists automatically send the information to the primary care physician. Therefore, it is imperative that you request in the strongest manner that the report be sent to your primary care physician as soon as possible (in a timely manner). It is possible that you might have to be seen by a number of specialists. The only physician who will have all of the medical information will be your primary care physician. He or she is your gatekeeper and your advocate in making sure that all treatments recommended by the specialists are compatible with each other and with your other medical conditions.

**Your primary care physician is the key
to ensuring you receive quality care.**

Chapter 3:
How to Communicate
with Your Physician

Being able to communicate with your physician is the most important aspect of your relationship. However, there are several things that you must do to assure that the communication is effective.

Let's focus first on the subject of health insurance. You should know your insurance company, the address, your policy number, and your deductible. It is best to have a card that you can show to the office staff; most likely the staff will copy the card and put the information in your file. This is your responsibility. It is your health insurance not theirs. Most physicians will submit the claim for you, but they need information. Do not ask them to waste their time finding out your information when you should do that long before the appointment. If you do not know what your policy covers, then call the insurance company and ask.

You must be a good historian. It is interesting that people make fun of patients who write down all of their illnesses, symptoms, or medications. This information is critical to the physician. History of hospitalizations, treatments, old X-rays (films and reports), CAT scans, MRIs, a list of medications, and old medical records should be forwarded from your previous physician to your new physician. A family history should be collected and a file created that can be copied and given to your primary care physician. The more information that a patient can provide to his or her physician, the more positive the outcome that will occur.

During that first get-acquainted appointment, you can learn what types of information your primary care physician will want. You need to make sure that you know the proper descriptive terms for symptoms and types of pain that you are experiencing. If there is a rule to follow about medical history information, it is that the information should be as complete and thorough as possible. This is not a game. Your life, in part, depends on this information. Unless you are incapacitated or incompetent, your medical information is your responsibility.

A form to help document your comprehensive history is included in appendix B under Medical History. This will help you collect your thoughts about your history and current symptoms or health complaints before you see the physician. When you speak to the physician, try to be accurate and articulate about your condition, i.e., type of pain, where the pain is located, tiredness, discomfort, etc. It is also important to report all allergies (food, medication, or environmental) and all medications that you are currently taking.

Many people have a great deal of difficulty talking to a physician. These individuals have such high anxiety that they actually develop physical symptoms, i.e., elevated blood pressure, shortness of breath, nausea, and loss of focus. If this is you, there is no need to be ashamed. In fact, it is quite normal. But, you still need to communicate with your physician. I suggest that you write everything down and take the document to the appointment. Record all of your symptoms (length, severity, and time of day), all medications, previous medical history (illnesses, surgery, and injuries), and allergies (food, pollen, dander, etc.).

Here are a few tips for preparing yourself to see the physician.

1. First and most importantly, take some slow deep breaths. Clear your mind and calm yourself.
2. Tell yourself that the physician is your friend and is there to help you.
3. Remember early diagnosis and intervention is very important.
4. Go over your written lists.
5. Have a family member or close friend go with you.
6. Try to think positive thoughts.

When the physician asks you what is wrong, you should give a concise, comprehensive report. He or she will give you an examination. It is possible that blood work or diagnostic-imaging tests will be ordered. It is important to ask what the tests are for and what the physician is considering as it relates to your condition. Questions are good.

Never, never feel that you shouldn't ask questions or that you ask too many questions.

You should never leave the physician's office until you fully understand the diagnosis and the treatment plan. If you feel that you cannot understand the diagnosis or the plan, then ask your family member/friend to join you and let the physician explain it to that person. It is imperative that you or someone close to you has a complete understanding of your condition and the treatment plan.

Going to see the physician and understanding what he or she says is a good first step. It is important that you follow the physician's orders. Noncompliance is a major contributor to the failure of patients to improve from a course of treatment. Let me give you some quick examples.

Your physician prescribes an antibiotic for the congestion in your chest and your sore throat. You are to take the medication for ten days, but you start feeling better on day five and stop taking the antibiotic. The problem comes back and is more severe than the original infection.

You are being **noncompliant**—not following your doctor's directions. This could lead to you not getting the full benefit of the prescribed treatment.

You have adult-onset diabetes. Your physician has told you to lose weight and reduce your sugar intake. You receive a diet from your physician's office, and the physician expects you to follow it. It has been explained to you that you must change your lifestyle or else you will have to take medication to control your blood sugar level. It has been explained to you that diabetes is not an insignificant illness, and you must lower your blood sugar or else other physical problems will occur. You follow the diet (sort of) for a couple of weeks, and then quit and go back to your old lifestyle. Your blood sugar level spikes, and your physician must put you on medication. **Noncompliance.**

You have been diagnosed with hypertension (high blood pressure). You have been told to lower your cholesterol by diet, stop all intake of salt, and lose weight. You do not comply, and the physician must put you on medication. **Noncompliance.**

If you are not going to comply with your physician's orders, then you are wasting your time and the physician's. If you trust your physician, and you communicate well with him or her, then follow his or her advice and move to a healthier future. One of the reasons that health care is getting more expensive is in part due to noncompliant patients. Most medications are very expensive. Life is too short to allow for poor health. It is not fair that you have a problem (but that's life), however, it would be even worse not to take care of it. As a rule, most health problems start out small and escalate to major complications if not treated. It's your choice.

The well-informed, well-prepared, and compliant patient will have better success in living long and prospering (as Mr. Spock used to say). You only have your health. Take your physician's advice seriously because your health is the most important thing in your life and your loved ones' lives.

Chapter 4:
Choosing a Health Insurance
Carrier and Type of Policy

In March of 2010, Congress passed the Health Care Reform Act (Reform Act). This legislation is more about access to and regulations that pertain to health insurance. There is very little in the act that affects the actual care delivered to the patient.

The new regulations make it more difficult for insurance companies to deny health insurance to an individual with preexisting medical conditions. Further, insurance companies cannot drop individuals from their coverage for utilization of the policy. The Reform Act deals mostly with access to health insurance and how the cost of that access will be paid.

The new act notwithstanding, health insurance is a very tricky area of health care. The number of insurance carriers and types of policies available can be overwhelming. Health care insurance is essentially based on one thing: money. The more comprehensive the policy, the more it will cost.

Before you look at different types of policies, I suggest that you evaluate two things: first, the state of your health and that of your family, and second, the state of your finances. You should take a hard look at your budget and determine whether you could financially afford a serious illness or condition.

Health insurance is usually paid by a monthly or quarterly premium. Obviously, you must calculate your monthly income. Each individual must determine the position of importance that health care has in his or her budget. It is important to remember that one hospitalization or long-term illness will have a crippling effect on your finances if you are not insured. Therefore, at the very least you should have some sort of hospitalization coverage. The Reform Act as passed by Congress requires that all Americans have health insurance.

Who can help?

You now have completed your analysis of your financial status and level of commitment to health care insurance. I recommend that you find an agent who has comprehensive knowledge of health care insurance policies. It would be better if this agent were employed by a multi-agent agency.

Larger firms usually have a larger menu of policy types to offer you. It is imperative that this agent acts as your advocate. The agent's approach should be to find the best policy for your medical and financial situation. If he or she is only interested in selling, move on to another agent. You should shop around and talk to family and friends about who they use and then meet the agent. The agent must be willing to assist you at all times with any policy questions or problems, and I am sure that you will have both.

When you have found a company and an agent that are acceptable to you, it is important that you go over a few scenarios when trying to pick the right type of policy. Pick a policy and imagine a hospitalization, long-term illness, or large number of outpatient diagnostic tests for you or a family member. Insist that the agent determine what your personal financial exposure would be based on the coverage of the policy that you are considering. This will give you some idea of what is covered, and what is not and how much it is going to cost you.

The Health Care Insurance Gamble

Eventually the question becomes **how much of a gambler are you?** Here are my thoughts on gambling with health care.

1. If you have a serious preexisting medical condition, you need a good comprehensive policy.
2. If you have children (they **will** get sick and require attention, and costs mount quickly), you will need a good family policy.
3. If you intend to have a child (prenatal care, labor, and delivery are very expensive), you need a good family policy. It is important to know whether the policy covers premature delivery and neonatal care.
4. If your job involves some sort of risk to your health, you need a good policy.

5. If your family history has a propensity for cardiovascular disease, hypertension, or any other disease, then you need a good policy.
6. If you are nineteen to twenty-seven years old and in good health, maybe your policy can be limited, but it must include hospitalization. This age range has a higher incidence of traffic accidents and sports injuries that might require a lengthy stay in a hospital.

New federal law will dictate what will be the minimum health insurance coverage allowed before a financial penalty is assessed to an individual.

Are you a gambler? If you become ill, the cost is astronomical and may bankrupt you in very short order. It is a question of priorities.

Types of Health Care Insurance

The types of health care insurance programs can be confusing. However, the programs can be described in five basic categories. The new Reform Act will use different combinations of these tried and tested standard policy types.

FOS	Traditional fee for service
PPO	Preferred provider organizations
PO	Point of service
EPO	Exclusive provider organizations
HMO	Health maintenance organizations

Traditional Fee for Service

Fee-for-service (indemnity) health coverage was the insurance standard for many years. Chances are this is the type of health insurance that your father had many years ago. This type of insurance allows the individual to see any physician or other health care providers and use any hospital. The insurance company does not require that the individual contact it for permission to see a specialist or receive medical care from a specific facility.

However, you do not have complete control. Most of the existing fee-for-service programs require clearance for things such as visiting an emergency room. Remember this:

An insurance company cannot dictate whom you see or where you go for treatment, but it can and will tell you that it will not pay for claims that fall outside its policy rules.

There are financial consequences to this freedom of choice. The deductible for this type of policy is usually no less than $200 per year per individual. Once you have met your deductible, the insurance will pay 80 percent of the bill. Sometimes you will have to pay the bill to the physician up front and submit a claim to the insurance company for reimbursement and sometimes the physician will submit the claim for you.

Like most insurance carriers, the company has created a fee schedule for medical expenses. It is called *usual and customary*. This means that the insurance company has looked at charges from other physicians or care providers in the region and determined the average fee. In the last ten years, this charge has been the lowest charge in the region and not the average. If your physician charges more than the usual and customary accepted charge of the insurance company, you will have to pay the difference.

So, fee for service gives you freedom of choice but at a higher out of pocket expense.

Interestingly, most physicians and hospitals have contracted with insurance companies for rates and services, and that makes the issue of freedom of choice somewhat moot.

Managed Care

Managed care has become synonymous with bad care or less care. Actually, managed care has been around for over seventy years. In the purest sense, managed care is a program where the insurance company has negotiated fee structures and rates with a specific list of health care providers or facilities. The policyholder uses one of the providers on the insurance company's list and receives a discounted fee or the cost is completely covered by the insurance company. Thus, the carrier has managed the cost.

Managed care is now an integral part of the administration of health care. Case management, disease management, utilization review, and most importantly outcome analysis are highly developed disciplines in the health care delivery industry. Each of these areas has made a difference in how care is delivered to the patient. Case management is highly effective in maintaining compliance with a patient treatment plan and reducing redundant testing.

Disease management has created a gold standard based on state of the art medical treatment protocols for the top ten diseases in this country. This gives the care provider, facilities, and the patient access to the most recent protocols for treatment of specific diseases.

Utilization review and outcome analysis focus on the success of the treatment plan and attempts to eliminate the poor or unsuccessful delivery or treatment. Preferred provider organization, point of service organization, exclusive provider organization, and health maintenance organizations all operate as managed care organizations.

Preferred Provider Organization (PPO)

PPOs have created a network of providers that have agreed to lower fees in exchange for being included in a very exclusive list. Policyholders are given a financial incentive to stay within the exclusive network. If you stay within the network, the PPO will cover the bill. However, if you go outside the network, you may have to pay upfront and submit the bill to the PPO. The PPO may only pay 80 percent of the bill, which leaves you holding a substantial payment to the provider. If you stay in the network, you can refer yourself to any specialist that is in the network, and if you go outside the network, you may have to pay a portion of or the entire bill. PPOs usually do not pay for preventive health care services.

Point of Service (POS)

POSs are really PPOs that require a gatekeeper, namely the primary care physician. Each policyholder must choose a primary care physician from the limited list of network primary care providers. However, the primary care physician must make referrals to specialists, and the specialists must be in the network. If the policyholder refers himself or herself in or out of the network, the cost to the policyholder will be greater. Interestingly, POSs usually cover preventive care and some health improvement programs.

Exclusive Provider Organization (EPO)

EPOs are PPOs that work like HMOs. The network is not very large, and if the policyholder goes outside the network, he or she is usually responsible for the entire bill.

Health Maintenance Organization (HMO)

HMOs are the least flexible and have the most closed panel of providers. This is a group plan and is usually not an individual policyholder's plan. The policyholder has a low premium and a low co-payment or no co-payment at all.

This lower cost is possible because the policyholder must stay in network, must have the primary care physician refer him or her to a network specialist, and usually needs prior clearance from the HMO for an emergency room visit.

HMOs have large facilities or networks of clinics like Kaiser Permanente or require the policyholder to see only network physicians. When the policyholder goes outside the network, he or she is responsible for the entire bill.

HMOs are usually in the forefront for preventive medicine and health improvement services. HMOs are less expensive but highly limited and subject to HMO clearance for certain services.

Health insurance is important to your medical and financial health and that of your family. As I stated earlier, a good health insurance agent who handles all these types of insurance is invaluable to you when you are deciding which type to purchase.

Chapter 5:
Getting a Second Opinion

I firmly believe in second opinions, especially if it involves the diagnosis of a serious illness such as cancer or the recommendation for major surgery.

Most, if not all, physicians will not be offended by a patient's desire for a second opinion. If your physician is offended or becomes surly when you indicate that you would like a second opinion, it is time to find another physician. Do not let yourself be bullied by the physician or the physician's staff. Stand your ground. Second opinions are not out of the ordinary.

Medicine is an art not an exact science. Physicians are, believe it or not, human. They can miss something, not put all of the data together for the right diagnosis, not know the most recent treatment program, not have similar experiences, or just be having a bad day. It is important for you to get another examination and the corresponding diagnosis.

Almost all insurance carriers cover second opinions. The second opinion should be acquired as quickly as possible after the initial diagnosis. Make certain that you go through the proper channels of your insurance carrier so that the opinion is covered. I cannot stress enough that you seek out a physician who is a specialist known for his or her extensive knowledge or technique relating to your condition to render your second opinion. However, if you go to a specialist for a second opinion and decide to use the specialist to treat you, I recommend that you do not go back to the original physician; stay with the second physician.

If it were a member of my family or me, I would want the best possible treatment plan determined by the most knowledgeable physician available.

Once again, your primary care physician can be of immense help in this area. He or she has knowledge of all the specialists in the region. Just as word of mouth is a powerful tool in marketing and sales, it is the same in medicine. Physicians will share their experiences with each other as it relates to professional interactions with other physicians. So, your primary care physician has the knowledge and can be of great assistance in this matter.

Chapter 6:
Diagnoses and Treatment Plans

The first five chapters of this book are dedicated to helping you find the right physician and right insurance policy. If you are diagnosed with an injury or serious illness, you will need diagnostic services.

Diagnostic Services

Radiology

Diagnostic radiology facilities are not all the same. Just like physical medicine is an art, so is reading an X-ray, CT, MRI, PET, mammography, or GI series. You must make sure that the facility has a good reputation for the specific study or machine that you require.

For example, if you have a cardiac condition, then you would want to go to a facility that has an expertise in cardiac imaging or if you have a condition involving the brain, you want to go to a facility that images the brain routinely both with CT, MRI, and PET. The radiologist must be board certified and have extensive experience in the imaging modality for which you are scheduled.

The new radiological imaging equipment usually requires that the patient be placed in a small closed-in area. In the case of CT, MRI, or PET, it is a small tunnel-like opening. Many good radiology technologists can talk you through the procedure. However, all these imaging systems are very intolerant of patient movement. If you are anxious about being enclosed, you are not alone—many patients feel the same way, so it is no cause for embarrassment. You have the right to receive medication to help you tolerate the closeness of the tunnel. It would be best to tell the radiology group at the time of scheduling that you are sensitive to enclosed areas and will need some type of medication to tolerate the test. If you choose to try the imaging procedure without medication and find that you cannot tolerate the closeness, you have the right to request that the procedure be stopped, you be removed from the machine, and the test rescheduled with medication. In the case of MRI, there is the so-called open-air magnet. It is a wonderful MRI for patients who just cannot tolerate the standard machine or who are too large to fit in the standard tunnel. However, I believe that the images are not as good as the large standard MRIs, especially for images of the brain. I must stress that you should get the study done in whichever way you can best tolerate. These images are critical to your diagnosis and treatment.

Importantly, I would want the best and most experienced radiologist reading my images. Further, I would get copies of the images and have another qualified radiologist who specialized in my condition for a second opinion. It is reasonable to expect that your primary care physician will assist you in this process.

Laboratory Services

Laboratory services include tissue pathology and blood analysis (cell counts and chemistry), urine, stool analysis, etc.

To perform blood work, laboratories must be certified by the state and federal government. In order for a lab to participate in Medicare, it must pass a laboratory assessment test. So, I am not as concerned with the specimen analysis of a lab as I am the interpretation of tissue biopsies by a pathologist. Once again, the pathologist should be board certified and have extensive experience examining tissue samples of the specific type of tumor, cancer, or growth that he or she is identifying. If the diagnosis were cancer or any other serious condition, I would instruct my surgeon to make certain that enough tissue is taken for at least two examinations. Further, I would want the lab to maintain the extra tissue in the proper manner so that it could be examined by another pathologist.

Here is an example of why a second opinion is so important. The patient has a very large abdominal mass (the size of a grapefruit). During exploratory surgery, the surgeon removes a tissue sample for pathological examination. The pathologist reports that the tissue is a very unusual type of cancer. The incidence of this cancer is so low and so rare that the pathologist has only seen one or two samples over his or her career. Upon hearing that it is an unusual cancer, I would want to know the pathologist's experience with this diagnosis. Regardless of his or her answer, I would insist that the tissue sample be sent to a pathologist that was an expert with this cancer. The first place that I would send the sample to would be the Armed Forces Institute of Pathology (AFIP) and its expert in this area. This happened to a member of my family. The patient was at a prominent teaching institution and this very unusual identification was made. The patient was pressured to have radiation therapy immediately. I insisted that the sample be sent to AFIP before any new treatment was performed. What was diagnosed by the teaching hospital as an unusual and deadly cancer was diagnosed by the expert at AFIP as a harmless fat tumor. Always insist on a second opinion. Arrogance is not limited to just politicians.

Navigating the Cancer Diagnosis

Let's use the diagnosis of breast cancer as an example of how one might navigate through this horrible ordeal. During self-examination of your breast, you feel a lump. Breast lumps usually appear in women but can occur in men. Obviously, this is very disturbing, but fortunately you have enough forethought to go see your primary care physician. The physician also feels the lump and schedules you for a mammogram. This physician knows which radiology center specializes in digital mammography. The radiologist who will read the study is well trained in the interpretation of digital mammography. Despite this radiologist's expertise, I would have the images read by another mammography expert.

Unfortunately, both radiologists see the same thing—breast cancer. The reports are sent to your primary care physician who then refers you to an oncologist. When conversing with your primary care physician about this referral, make sure that this specialist has extensive experience in the treatment of breast cancer. I would make sure your primary care physician knows that regardless of the outcome of your visit to the oncologist, you will want a second opinion.

Each oncologist will examine you and present a diagnosis and a treatment plan. The oncologist will order a tissue biopsy that confirms the existence of cancer. Before you decide on which plan to accept, you should go over both plans with your primary care physician. The two of you should discuss the plans and decide which one to follow. Together you might decide that the best plan is chemotherapy, followed by surgery, and then radiation therapy.

Obviously, you want to go to the best chemotherapy unit in your area. You want this unit to have a high rate of success and an even higher level of compassion for its patients. Besides the technical competency of the chemo unit, it is important for the attending physician and the staff to educate you on what is going to happen technically and to your body.

You are likely going to lose your hair and have intense nausea. During the course of the treatment, you are going to be exhausted and possibly depressed. If any of these conditions become overwhelming, you must call the physician delivering the chemotherapy and your primary care physician. There are medications that can help. I would keep my primary care physician in the information loop at all times. He or she is your gatekeeper: the only physician who has all of the information concerning your condition and past health. Your primary care physician is a wonderful and important resource during this ordeal.

So now you have finished your chemo, and the latest mammogram shows that the cancer is gone. Do not believe it. Stay the course of the treatment plan. Surgery is very important to the survival of breast cancer. Mastectomy, whether partial or radical, is critical to your survival. It requires that you find the right surgeon. There are multiple techniques for a mastectomy. It is important that you discuss the technique with your surgeon and agree on the one that suits you best. If you and the surgeon do not agree on the technique, find another surgeon.

One important note, you should discuss the number of lymph nodes that the surgeon will take as samples for pathology. I recommend that you ask for primary, secondary, and tertiary lymph node biopsies.

Breast cancer treatment is not easy. The patient is exhausted, nauseous, in pain from the surgery, and possibly depressed. The first two components of the treatment plan may stretch over as many as three months. This is a very long time to keep your spirits up and maintain your resolve to finish the program. Nevertheless, radiation therapy is critical to the success of the total treatment plan. Radiation therapy is relatively painless, but emotionally and physically draining over the course of the long treatment plan. Stay the course. Family and friends must come to your aid to help you through this ordeal. Thankfully, there are some wonderful web pages to assist the patient with information and counseling. (See appendix A for listing)

After the radiation therapy, you will be given a schedule of times for visits to the oncologist, the surgeon, and your primary care physician. It is absolutely imperative that you keep these appointments. Your life depends on this.

This example demonstrates the need for communication, using facilities and physicians that have the proper training and expertise, and keeping your primary care physician in the loop. Commitment, courage, and the love of family and friends will help you through this ordeal.

The Cardiovascular Scenario

Another example of treatment plans and diagnoses is that of cardiovascular disease. You might call this hardening of the arteries, high blood pressure, or even heart attack. This scenario starts in the primary care physician's office. You present yourself with shortness of breath, chest pain radiating down your left arm, and/or a strange feeling in your chest. The physician performs an EKG on you, and it is abnormal.

If it is determined that your condition is life threatening, your physician will send you to the hospital emergency room. If it is not life threatening, your physician will refer you to a cardiologist. After the cardiologist's examination, it is determined that you might have blockage of the coronary arteries of your heart (the arteries that feed your heart). You are scheduled for a stress and myocardial perfusion test. I recommend that a board certified nuclear cardiologist perform this study.

You will be asked to walk or jog on a treadmill to get your heart rate up to the maximum predicted rate or to *stress* it; then a harmless radioactive solution will be injected into you. This radioactive solution has a propensity to go to healthy cardiac cells. This study will show the areas of the heart that are not receiving enough blood. Each area of the heart is served by a specific coronary artery. So, the nuclear cardiologist will be able to determine which vessels are blocked.

If the study is abnormal, you may be scheduled for cardiac catheterization. I would want to be catheterized by a physician who has extensive experience in this procedure. During this procedure, a catheter is run from the groin to the heart, and a dye is injected into each coronary artery. X-rays are taken that show how much, if any, of the dye is progressing through each of the coronary arteries. The physician can calculate the amount of blockage in each vessel. Based on the results of this study, the cardiologist, the primary care physician, and you will decide the proper course of treatment.

A new procedure employs medicated stents. The stent is placed into the vessel at the point of blockage, and the vessel is opened for blood to flow to the heart tissues that the vessel serves. If the stent is not appropriate, then coronary bypass surgery may be required. This is major life-threatening surgery. The traditional surgery requires that the cardiac surgeon open the chest to get access to the heart. Veins from the legs are harvested and grafted on to the blocked vessel to bypass the blockage and restore blood flow.

Obviously, you want the cardiac surgeon (heart surgeon) to have a great deal of experience and a high rate of success. I would make sure that the hospital also has an excellent reputation for cardiac surgery. The use of stents or the cardiac surgery has significant risk. It is imperative that you, your cardiologist, the cardiac surgeon, and your primary care physician be involved in this plan.

Both of these scenarios are serious health problems. As a patient, you cannot eliminate all the risk. But with good communication, good facilities, and good physicians you can minimize the risk and assure a more successful outcome.

Chapter 7:
Hospitals and You

Charles Dickens wrote: "It was the best of times, it was the worst of times." Hospitals are the best of places for treatment, but hospitals are the worst of places for infections. Not all hospitals are created equal. Teaching hospitals, such as universities, are huge. In a large teaching hospital, you will be treated by your attending or a hospital physician. However, because it is a teaching institution, the physician's interns or residents will also see you. They used to be called *ducklings* because they follow the momma or papa duck (physician) around during medical rounds. Large teaching hospitals are wonderful for exotic diseases, new cutting-edge or experimental treatments, and new surgical techniques. However, if your medical condition can be accommodated in a community-based hospital, I recommend that you use the smaller facility. In a community-based hospital, infection control is more effective and successful. The number of physicians poking and prodding you is limited to just your attending physician. This reduces the number of chances for miscommunication and repeated examinations. You and your family can maintain some control in a smaller facility. Obviously, physicians need to be trained in teaching facilities, but this book is about you and what is best for you as the patient.

When you are going to be treated in a hospital, you must focus on how to protect yourself while you're there. You must surround yourself with as many advocates as possible. Your attending physician should be your primary advocate and must make sure that all his or her medical orders are followed to the letter and that no other orders are followed unless authorized by him or her. The attending must make sure that the patient is not given any *misadministrations.*

A *misadministration* means that the patient was given the wrong treatment, medication, diagnostic test, or surgical procedure. For example, several years ago in a hospital in Florida a patient had the wrong leg amputated. After a great deal of finger-pointing and hospital promises of improving proper surgical identification, the hospital repeated the mistake with another patient.

The number of misadministrations across this country has increased exponentially in the last ten years. This is an alarming situation that is unknown to the public. As a patient you must protect yourself; if you are conscious and coherent, you must ask questions: name and purpose of each medication you are given, where are you being taken, and what test is to be performed.

When it comes to surgery, you must make certain that you are properly identified (for all to see) and that the type of surgery you are going to have performed by the surgeon is clear to everyone. However, the patient is not always well enough to protect him or herself. This is where the family is so important. I recommend that there be a family member with the patient at all times. Each family member must know the treatment plan. It is important to organize this effort so that all family members who are going to stand guard are present when the attending physician speaks to the family to outline the treatment plan.

When the family member asks the physician questions, it's important to let him or her know that the family is concerned about the care delivered by the hospital and wants to protect the patient from any misadministrations. The physician should go over his or her orders related to medications, treatments, and diagnostic tests.

Armed with this information, a family member has a good chance of stopping a misadministration before it occurs. If the staff of the hospital gives you a hard time, call your attending and ask the physician to intercede and speak directly to the staff. If the attending will not do this, call patient relations and ask for help; then find another attending physician. The attending physician's only concern should be the patient, and he or she should realize what the family member is trying to accomplish. Your attending physician should be your most important advocate.

If a misadministration does occur, regardless of the severity of the mistake, call your legal counsel. Do not let the hospital administration bully you or seduce you into giving up your legal rights. You should insist that you will not speak to any hospital official unless your legal counsel is present. It appears that the only way that this epidemic of misadministrations is going to end is if the public insists that hospitals accept responsibility for their actions.

I hate medical lawsuits. These suits are a major reason for the incredible increase in health care costs. However, it appears that until the industry starts correcting these issues in a comprehensive manner, it is the only protection the public has from this type of negligence.

My philosophy is that the squeaky wheel gets the grease. I recommend that you squeak loudly but respectfully. You should make sure that your complaints are legitimate and fair. The complaints should be about the care that is delivered and not about something frivolous. I am not against hospitals. This book is about how the patient deals with the health care industry. Hospitals are well acquainted with how to protect themselves. According to a new study published in the *Archives of Internal Medicine*[1], 48,000 people died from hospital-acquired infections in 2006. One must always be on guard.

If you are a patient who has been treated by a specialist in the hospital, you must make sure that the specialist speaks to your primary care physician about your stay and the proposed follow-up treatment plan

---

1   Michael R. Eber, Ramanan Laxminarayan, Eli N. Perencevich, et al., **"Clinical and Economic Outcomes Attributable to Health Care–Associated Sepsis and Pneumonia," Arch. Intern. Med. 170, 4 (2010): 347-353.**

devised by the specialist. It would be smart to have the specialist send a copy of your pertinent medical records concerning your hospitalization and the treatment plan to your primary care physician. Remember, the primary care physician is the gatekeeper. He or she is the only physician who has a complete picture of your medical condition.

Chapter 8:
Health Care Confusion

This chapter is dedicated to some of the confusion, misconceptions, and health care myths.

The common cold: Antibiotics do not cure the common cold. In fact, nothing effectively cures the common cold. A virus causes the common cold. All the drugs that the doctor gives you or that you buy over the counter are for the relief of symptoms from the common cold not for its cure. However, antibiotics will assist in combating any bacterial infection that may occur from the cold. So, if your physician gives you antibiotics and tells you to take them for ten days, please follow his or her orders. When your physician tells you to get rest, keep hydrated (drink lots of fluids), and keep quiet until your body has time to fight off the cold, I strongly suggest that you comply with your physician's instructions.

My insurance company will not let me go to that physician or have that test or be given that treatment. Let me make this as clear and direct as I can: an insurance company cannot tell you what to do. The only thing that an insurance company can do is tell you what your policy will cover and not cover, which physician is or is not in their network, and what treatments are eligible for coverage and which are not. You and your physician decide what is needed for your medical condition. If the insurance company refuses to pay for it, and your physician feels that it is medically necessary, then you have the right to challenge the insurance company and have the denial reviewed by its medical affairs committee that handles these requests. I recommend that you and your physician prepare a short written narrative explaining why the request is medically necessary and make sure that it is entered into the file in front of this committee. I would also send a letter to the insurance commissioner of your state that details the problem and includes the short narrative that you and your physician prepared. I would send a copy of this letter to the insurance company's medical review committee. This lets the committee know that you are serious and cannot be easily dismissed. If you can afford it, legal counsel is very helpful. If you and your physician feel that this is very important to your care, then stand your ground. I am absolutely sure that initially the insurance company will ignore you and then attempt to intimidate you. Stand your ground. Demand that your situation be heard and that the insurance company cover your care.

I cannot see my medical records. Nonsense. They are records about you. You have the right to see them. The federal law called the Health Insurance Portability and Accountability Act of 1996 Privacy Rule (HIPPA) gives you the right to see and get copies of your medical records. HIPPA requires that all health care providers and their business agents must protect your medical records and keep them private. The government Web site www.hhs.gov describes HIPPA and the federal regulations that protect your medical records. You have the right to see and copy the original records, but you will have to pay for the copies of the records (the fees must be reasonable). This includes all medical records (except psychotherapy notes or information compiled for litigation or if the provider can prove that the information will harm you or someone else), reports, radiology images, and billing and appointment logs. Further, you have the right to expect that all health care providers and their agents will maintain your records in a secure and confidential manner. Each health care provider must certify that all records are secure and not available to the public. In addition, you must authorize the release of your medical records in writing in order for a provider to share them with other providers. Why is this so important? Your confidential medical records could affect your job or future jobs, health and life insurance policies, and your financial status. Your privacy is a very important issue to your life and family, so take it seriously and protect it.

The law says that I must sign up for Medicare when I am sixty-five.

Many of my friends are sixty-five or soon will be sixty-five. I get a lot of questions about Medicare—questions about signing up for Medicare and the difference between Part A and Part B.

Federal law does not require you to sign up for Medicare when you turn sixty-five.

47

You have the right to purchase any health care insurance policy that fits your needs. However, not signing up with Medicare creates a major issue. **If you do not sign up with Medicare when you turn sixty-five and then decide to take Medicare later, there is a penalty (increase in fees) associated with that decision.** Obviously, except for very unique circumstances, I recommend that you enroll in the Medicare Part A and Part B and purchase Medicare supplemental insurance (sometimes called MediGap), which will cover the expenses that Medicare Part A and B do not.

The monthly premium charged by Medicare for Part B depends on the amount of income that you report on your Internal Revenue Tax returns; obviously, the higher your income, the higher the monthly premium. Presently (2010), the highest monthly premium is $353.60.

In the appendix, chapter 8: Health Care Confusion, you will find a short discussion on Medicare Part A and Part B.

Chapter 9:
Take Control!

The intention of this book is to encourage you to take control of your life as it relates to your health care. Communication, the willingness to become actively involved in your health care, and the resolve to correct what is not correct or appealing to you are the keys to navigating the American health care system.

Insisting that you be treated with respect, compassion, and intelligence will help you develop the interactive relationships that you will need with the physicians who care for you. Understanding that you must participate in your health care is critical to a healthy life. The willingness to research and understand your condition or the physician who is attending you will make the process work more effectively. Timidity will not help you obtain good health care. Instead, it is possible that it will cause you health problems.

The squeaky wheel gets the grease. When you are respectful and fair but demand the best possible care, you will get the grease. A passive attitude will very possibly bring you mediocre care, misadministrations, and certainly larger and inaccurate bills. It is my opinion that America has become timid. It appears that we are willing to accept poor service, mistakes, and disrespect; I think it has something to do with political correctness. Not me. I expect each and every person to do his or her job to the best of his or her ability. I expect each person to have the proper attitude. I expect to be treated with respect. When I am not treated properly, then I govern myself accordingly. I become "squeaky," but I temper it with respect and fairness. Nevertheless, I will be treated properly, or the offender will hear about it. My life depends on the proper care.

The responsibility for effectively navigating the health care system is yours; make the commitment and take control of your life!

APPENDIX A - References

References are provided by chapter; not all chapters have references.

References for Chapter 1 - Web Page References

Radiological Society of North America
www.rsna.org

American College of Radiology
www.acr.org

Pharmaceutical Research And Manufacturers of America
www.pharma.org

American Cancer Society
www.cancer.org

References for Chapter 2 - Physician Databases

American Medical Association
www.ama-assn.org

State Medical Licensing Boards
(see list beginning on page 56)

Physician Quality Reporting Initiative
www.medicare.org

American Board of Medical Specialties
www.abms.org

American Academy of Family Physicians
www.aafp.org

American College of Physicians
www.acponline.org

References for Chapter 4 - Health Insurance Carriers

Top Health Insurance Companies – U.S. News list of Best Health Plans
health.usnews.com/sections/health/health-plans/index.html

National Association of Insurance Commissioners
www.naic.org

References for Chapter 6 - Diagnostic Laboratory Certifications

Department of Health, Office of Health Care Quality for each state

Navigating the Cancer Diagnosis

Cancer Information Web Pages
   American Cancer Society www.cancer.org
   National Cancer Institute – Cancer Information Service www.cis.nci.nih.gov
   BreastCancer.org www.breastcancer.org
   Susan G. Komen for the Cure www.komen.org

Cardiovascular Diagnosis and Disease

American Heart Association   www.americanheart.org

Cardiovascular Disease Foundation www.cvdf.org

National Institute for Health - National Heart, Lung, & Blood Institute www.nhlb.nih.gov

References for Chapter 7
– Hospitals and You

Agency for Health Care Research and Quality - Medical Errors and Patient Safety www.ahrq.gov

Patient Advocacy
National Patient Advocate Foundation   www.npaf.org

State Medical Licensure Boards

Alabama State Board of Medical Examiners
848 Washington Ave
PO Box 946
Montgomery, AL 36101-0946
(334) 242-4116
(334) 242-4155 Fax
www.albme.org

Alaska State Medical Board
Division of Occupational Licensing
550 W Seventh Ave, Ste 1500
Anchorage, AK 99501
(907) 269-8163
(907) 269-8196 Fax
www.dced.state.ak.us/occ/pmed.htm

Arizona Medical Board
9545 E Doubletree Ranch Rd
Scottsdale, AZ 85258-5514
(480) 551-2700
(480) 551-2704 Fax
www.azmd.gov

Arkansas State Medical Board
2100 Riverfront Dr
Little Rock, AR 72202-1793
(501) 296-1802
(501) 603-3555
www.armedicalboard.org

Medical Board of California
2005 Evergreen St, Ste 1200
Sacramento, CA 95815
(916) 263-2389
(916) 263-2387 Fax
www.medbd.ca.gov

Colorado Board of Medical Examiners
1560 Broadway, Ste 1300
Denver, CO 80202-5140
(303) 894-7690
(303) 894-7692 Fax
www.dora.state.co.us/medical

Connecticut Medical Examining Board
Physician Licensure Unit
PO Box 340308, 410 Capital Ave, MS 13PHO
Hartford, CT 06134-0308
(860) 509-7648
(860) 509-7553 Fax
www.dph.state.ct.us

Delaware Board of Medical Examiners
861 Silver Lake Blvd, Ste 203
Cannon Building
Dover, DE 19904
(302) 744-4500
(302) 739-2711 Fax
www.dpr.delaware.gov

District of Columbia Board of Medicine
Health Professional Licensing Administration
717 14th St NW, Rm 1007
Washington, DC 20005
(202) 724-8800
(202) 727-8471 Fax
www.dchealth.dc.gov

Florida Board of Medicine
Bin #C03
4052 Bald Cypress Way
Tallahassee, FL 32399-3253
(850) 245-4131
(850) 488-9325 Fax
www.doh.state.fl.us

Georgia Composite State Board of Medical Examiners
2 Peachtree St NW, 36th Floor
Atlanta, GA 30303
(404) 656-3913
(404) 656-9723 Fax
www.medicalboard.state.ga.us

Guam Board of Medical Examiners
651 Legacy Square Commercial Complex
S Route 10, Ste 9
Marfilao, GU 96913
(671) 735-7406
(671) 735-7413 Fax

Hawaii Board of Medical Examiners
335 Merchant St, Rm 301

PO Box 3469
Honolulu, HI 96813
(808) 586-2689
(808) 586-2874 Fax
www.ehawaii.gov

Idaho State Board of Medicine
1755 Westgate Dr, Ste 140
Boise, ID 83704
(208) 327-7000
(208) 327-7005 Fax
www.bom.state.id.us

Illinois Medical Licensing Board
Department of Professional Regulation
320 W Washington, 3rd Floor
Springfield, IL 62786
(217) 557-3209
(217) 524-2169
www.idfpr.com

Medical Licensing Board of Indiana
402 W Washington St, Rm W072
Indianapolis, IN 46204
(317) 234-2060
(317) 233-4236 Fax
www.in.gov/pla/medical.htm

Iowa Board of Medical Examiners
400 SW 8th St, Ste C
Des Moines, IA 50309-4686
(515) 281-6641

(515) 242-5908 Fax
www.medicalboard.iowa.gov

Kansas Board of Healing Arts

235 S Topeka Blvd
Topeka, KS 66603-3068
(785) 296-8561
(785) 296-0852 Fax
www.ksbha.org

Kentucky Board of Medical Licensure

Hurstbourne Office Park
310 Whittington Pkwy, Ste 1B
Louisville, KY 40222-4916
(502) 429-7150
(502) 429-7158 Fax
http://kbml.ky.gov

Louisiana State Board of Medical Examiners

630 Camp St
PO Box 30250
New Orleans, LA 70190-0250
(504) 568-6820 x262
(504) 568-8893 Fax
www.lsbme.org

Maine Board of Licensure in Medicine

161 Capitol St
137 State House Station
Augusta, ME 04333
(207) 287-3601
(207) 287-6590 Fax
www.docboard.org/me/me_home.htm

Maryland Board of Physicians
PO Box 2571
4201 Patterson Ave, 4th Floor
Baltimore, MD 21215-0095
(410) 764-4777
(410) 358-2252 Fax
www.mbp.state.md.us

Massachusetts Board of Registration in Medicine
560 Harrison Ave, Ste G-4
Boston, MA 02118
(617) 654-9800
(617) 451-9568 Fax
www.massmedboard.org

Michigan Board of Medicine
611 W Ottawa St, 1st Floor
PO Box 30670
Lansing, MI 48933
(517) 373-6873
(517) 373-2179
www.michigan.gov/healthlicense

Minnesota Board of Medical Practice
University Park Plaza 2829 University Ave SE, Ste 400
Minneapolis, MN 55414-3246
(612) 617-2130
(612) 617-2166 Fax
www.bmp.state.mn.us

Mississippi State Board of Medical Licensure

1867 Crane Ridge Dr, Ste 200B
Jackson, MS 39216
(601) 987-3079
(601) 987-4159 Fax
www.msbml.state.ms.us

Missouri State Board of Registration for the Healing Arts

Division of Professional Registration
3605 Missouri Blvd
Jefferson City, MO 65109
(573) 751-0098
(573) 751-3166 Fax
www.pr.mo.gov/healingarts.asp

Montana Board of Medical Examiners

PO Box 200513
301 S Park Ave, 4th Floor
Helena, MT 59620-0513
(406) 841-2364
(406) 841-2343 Fax
www.discoveringmontana.com/dli/bsd/license/
bsd_boards/
med_board/board_page.asp

Nebraska Board of Medicine and Surgery

Regulation and Licensure Credentialing Division
301 Centennial Mall South, PO Box 94986
Lincoln, NE 68509-4986
(402) 471-2118
(402) 471-3577 Fax
www.hhs.state.ne.us

Nevada State Board of Medical Examiners
1105 Terminal Way, Ste 301
Reno, NV 89502
(775) 688-2559
(775) 688-2321 Fax
www.medboard.nv.gov

New Hampshire Board of Medicine
2 Industrial Park Dr, Ste 8
Concord, NH 03301-8520
(603) 271-1205
(603) 271-6702 Fax
www.state.nh.us/medicine

New Jersey State Board of Medical Examiners
PO Box 183
140 E Front St, 2nd Floor
Trenton, NJ 08625-0183
(609) 826-7100
(609) 826-7117 Fax
www.state.nj.us/lps/ca/medical.htm

New Mexico Medical Board
2055 S Pacheco St
Building 400
Santa Fe, NM 87505
(505) 476-7221
(505) 476-7233
www.state.nm.us/nmbme

New York State Board of Medicine
89 Washington Ave
2nd Floor, West Wing
Albany, NY 12234
(518) 474-3817 x560
(518) 486-4846 Fax
www.op.nysed.gov

North Carolina Medical Board
1203 Front St
PO Box 20007
Raleigh, NC 27619
(919) 326-1100 ext 218
(919) 326-1131 Fax
www.ncmedboard.org

North Dakota State Board of Medical Examiners
418 E Broadway Ave, Ste 12
Bismarck, ND 58501
(701) 328-6500
(701) 328-6505 Fax
www.ndbomex.com

State Medical Board of Ohio
30 E Broad St, 3rd Floor
Columbus, OH 43215-6127
(614) 466-3934
(614) 728-5946 Fax
www.med.ohio.gov

Oklahoma State Board of Medical Licensure and Supervision

PO Box 18256

Oklahoma City, OK 73154-0256

(405) 848-6841

(405) 848-4999 Fax

www.okmedicalboard.org

Oregon Board of Medical Examiners

1500 SW First Ave

620 Crown Plaza

Portland, OR 97201-5826

(503) 229-5770

(503) 229-6543 Fax

www.bme.state.or.us

Pennsylvania State Board of Medicine

2601 North Third St

PO Box 2649

Harrisburg, PA 17105-2649

(717) 783-1400

(717) 787-7769 Fax

www.dos.state.pa.us/bpoa

Board of Medical Examiners of Puerto Rico

PO Box 13969

San Juan, PR 00908

(787) 782-8949 or 782-8937

(787) 792-4436 Fax

Rhode Island Board of Medical Licensure and Discipline
Cannon Bldg, Rm 205
Three Capitol Hill
Providence, RI 02908-5097
(401) 222-3855
(401) 222-2158 Fax
www.health.ri.gov/hsr/bmld

South Carolina Board of Medical Examiners
Department of Labor, Licensing & Regulation
110 Centerview Dr, Ste 202
Columbia, SC 29210-1289
(803) 896-4500
(803) 896-4515 Fax
www.llr.state.sc.us/pol/medical

South Dakota State Board of Medical and Osteopathic Examiners
125 S Main Ave
Sioux Falls, SD 57104
(605) 367-7781
(605) 367-7786 Fax
www.state.sd.us/dcr/medical

Tennessee Board of Medical Examiners
227 French Landing #300
Nashville, TN 37243
(615) 532-3202
(615) 253-4484 Fax
www.state.tn.us/health

Texas State Board of Medical Examiners
PO Box 2018
Austin, TX 78768-2018
(512) 305-7010
(512) 305-7008 Fax
www.tmb.state.tx.us

Utah Department of Commerce
Division of Occupational & Professional Licensure
Heber M Wells Building, 4th Floor, 160 East 300
South
Salt Lake City, UT 84114-6741
(801) 530-6621
(801) 530-6511 Fax
www.dopl.utah.gov

Vermont Board of Medical Practice
108 Cherry St
PO Box 70
Burlington, VT 05402-0070
(802) 657-4220
(802) 657-4227 Fax
http://healthvermont.gov/hc/med_board/bmp.aspx

Virginia Board of Medicine
9960 Mayland Dr, Ste 300
Henrico, VA 23233-1463
(804) 367-4600
(804) 527-4426 Fax
www.dhp.virginia.gov

Virgin Islands Board of Medical Examiners
Office of the Commissioner, Department of Health
48 Sugar Estate
St Thomas, VI 00802
(340) 774-0117
(340) 777-4001 Fax

Washington Medical Quality Assurance Commission
Department of Health
PO Box 47866
Olympia, WA 98504-7866
(360) 236-4790
(360) 236-4573 Fax
www.doh.wa.gov

West Virginia Board of Medicine
101 Dee Dr
Charleston, WV 25311
(304) 558-2921 x 227
(304) 558-2084 Fax
www.wvdhhr.org/wvbom

State of Wisconsin Medical Examining Board
Dept of Regulation & Licensing
PO Box 8935
Madison, WI 53703-8935
(608) 266-2112
(608) 267-3816 Fax
http://drl.wi.gov

Wyoming Board of Medicine
320 W 25th St, Ste 103
Cheyenne, WY 82002
(307) 778-7053
(307) 778-2069
http://wyomedboard.state.wy.us

Arizona Board of Osteopathic Medical Examiners
9535 E Doubletree Ranch Rd
Scottsdale, AZ 85258-5539
(480) 657-7703 x22
(480) 657-7715 Fax
www.azdo.gov

Osteopathic Medical Board of California
1300 National Drive, #150
Sacramento, CA 95834
(916) 263-3100
(916) 263-3117 Fax
www.ombc.ca.gov

Florida Board of Osteopathic Medicine
Bin #C06
4052 Bald Cypress Way
Tallahassee, FL 32399-1753
(850) 245-4161
(850) 487-9874 Fax
www.doh.state.fl.us/mqa

Maine Board of Osteopathic Licensure
142 State House Station
Augusta, ME 04333-0142
(207) 287-2480
(207) 287-3015 Fax
www.maine.gov/osteo

Michigan Board of Osteopathic Medicine and Surgery
611 W Ottawa St, 1st Floor
Lansing, MI 48933
(517) 373-6873
(517) 373-2179 Fax
www.michigan.gov/healthlicense

Nevada State Board of Osteopathic Medicine
2860 E Flamingo Rd, Ste D
Las Vegas, NV 89121
(702) 732-2147
(702) 732-2079 Fax
www.osteo.state.nv.us

New Mexico Board of Osteopathic Medical Examiners
2550 Cerrillos Road
Santa Fe, NM 87505
(505) 476-4695
(505) 476-7095 Fax
www.rld.state.nm.us

Oklahoma Board of Osteopathic Examiners
4848 N Lincoln Blvd, Ste 100
Oklahoma City, OK 73105-3321
(405) 528-8625
(405) 557-0653 Fax
www.docboard.org

Pennsylvania State Board of Osteopathic Medicine
PO Box 2649
Harrisburg, PA 17101
(717) 783-4858
(717) 787-7769 Fax
www.dos.state.pa.us

Tennessee State Board of Osteopathic Examiners
First Floor Cordell Hull Bldg
425 5th Ave North
Nashville, TN 37247-1010
(615) 741-4540
(615) 253-4484 Fax
www.state.tn.us/health

State of Utah Department of Commerce
Division of Occupational & Professional Licensing
PO Box 146741
Salt Lake City, UT 84114-6741
(801) 530-6621
(801) 530-6511 Fax
www.dopl.utah.gov

Vermont Board of Osteopathic Physicians and Surgeons

Office of Professional Regulation
National Life Building, North Floor 2
Montpelier, VT 05620-3402
(802) 828-2367
(802) 828-2465
www.sec.state.vt.us

Washington Board of Osteopathic Medicine and Surgery

Department of Health
PO Box 47870
Olympia, WA 98504-7866
(360) 236-4943
(360) 236-2406 Fax
www.doh.wa.gov

West Virginia Board of Osteopathy

334 Penco Rd
Weirton, WV 26062
(304) 723-4638
(304) 723-2877 Fax
www.wvbdosteo.org

References for Chapter 8:
Health Care Confusion

Often I am asked what Medicare Part A covers and what Part A does not cover. Below is a short outline of covered items.

Medicare Part A helps pay for care in the following **facilities** if they are medically necessary (based on Medicare requirements), and you are eligible for Medicare Part A.

Medicare Part A Covered Facilities
- Inpatient care in hospitals (including critical access hospitals)
- Skilled nursing facilities (SNFs)
- Long-term care hospital (LTCH)
- Inpatient Rehabilitation Facility (IRF)
- Hospice care
- Home health care
- Beneficiary access to religious nonmedical health care institution (RNHCI) services
- Inpatient mental health/psychiatric care
- Obesity bariatric surgery

Medicare Part A also helps pay for the following services if they are medically necessary based on Medicare requirements. You must be eligible for Medicare Part A in order to get the following services.

Medicare Part A Covered Services

- Anesthesia
- Chemotherapy
- Health Care Facility's Room and Board
- All meals and special diets
- General nursing
- Medical social services
- Physical, occupational, and speech-language therapy
- Drugs with the exception of some self-administered drugs
- Blood transfusions
- Other diagnostic and therapeutic items and services
- Medical supplies and use of equipment
- Respite care in hospice
- Transportation services
- Inpatient alcohol or substance abuse treatment
- Part A blood (see the restrictions under noncovered services)
- Clinical trials (inpatient)
- Kidney dialysis (inpatient)

Medicare Part A Non-covered Services
Medicare Part A **DOES NOT** cover the following:

- Private duty nursing
- A television or telephone in your room or personal care items like razors, slippers, or socks
- A private room, unless medically necessary
- Custodial care, assisted living, adult day care, or reimbursement for family members
- The first three pints of blood unless the blood deductible has been met

The physician services you get while you are in a hospital may be filed under Part B.

Medicare Part B-Covered Services

Medicare B covers the physician services and other outpatient services (this is not an official or complete list)

Ambulance services
Ambulatory surgical centers
Blood services
Bone mass measurements
Cardiovascular services and screening
Chiropractic services
Clinical laboratory services
Colorectal cancer screening
Diabetes screening
Durable medical equipment
Emergency room services
Flu shots
Eye screening and services
Hearing examinations
Home health services
Kidney dialysis services
Mammograms service and screening
Mental health care
Nonphysician provider services
Occupation therapy
Outpatient hospital services and supplies
Pathological screening
Physical therapy
Prostate cancer screening
Prosthetic/orthotics equipment and services

Second surgical opinion
Speech: language pathology services
Radiological testing
Transplants and immunosuppressive drugs

But Medicare does not cover every test or service.

What is not covered by Part A or Part B?

If you need certain services that Medicare doesn't cover, you will have to pay out of pocket unless you have other insurance to cover the costs. Even if Medicare covers a service or item, you generally have to pay deductibles, coinsurance, and co-payments.

Items and services that Medicare does not cover include but are not limited to: long-term care, routine dental care, dentures, cosmetic surgery, acupuncture, hearing aids, and exams for fitting hearing aids. By no means should you consider these lists as complete, up to date, or official. They are supplied as guides to assist you in preparation for your conversation with an official Medicare representative.

To find out if Medicare covers a service you need, visit www.medicare.gov and select Find Out What Medicare Covers or call 1-800-MEDICARE (1-800-633-4227). TTY users should call 1-877-486-2048.

All of the Part A and Part B coverage information can be found in the Medicare Handbook called *Medicare & You.* This is a well-written handbook that you can get by downloading it from the Web page Medicare.gov or by calling Medicare and requesting that a copy be sent to you (1-800-medicare). Medicare has some wonderful booklets that will answer your questions.

Medicare & You

2009 Choosing A Medigap Policy: A Guide To Health Insurance For People With Medicare

Women and Heart Disease

Guide to Choosing a Nursing Home

Your Medicare Benefits

Call the 800-Medicare number and talk to well-trained staff. They can help you with all of your questions. If you have Web access, the medicare.gov Web page is very helpful.

Take charge and get answers!

Appendix B – Forms

Your Prescription List

Record each of your prescriptions below. Information can be found on the bottle. Take a copy of this list to the doctor's office each time you visit. Once you stop taking a prescription, draw a line through the entry.

Date Prescribed	Drug Name	Strength	Quantity	Directions	Expiration Date	Number of Refills

How to Navigate American Health Care – Forms

Date Prescribed	Drug Name	Strength	Quantity	Directions	Expiration Date	Number of Refills

Your Medical History

Family, Past, Most Recent Testing, Current Symptoms History Forms

Forms, forms, forms...you have to fill out forms everywhere. The forms in this section will make life so much easier for you in the long run. Yes, it is a tedious and time-consuming task to fill them out. However, having them completed will improve your communication with your physician and just might save your life or a loved one's life. Fill the forms out completely and ensure that they are accurate. If these forms are accurate and complete, they will be a wonderful resource that will repay you many times over.

Your Health History

Circle any items that apply to you that are out of the ordinary, persistent, or significant complaints. Use your common sense when completing this section

General and Head/Neck

Fever, Sweats, Chills	Eye Infections	Cavities
Weight Gain	Conjunctivitis	Dentures: Upper, Lower, Partials
Sudden Weight Loss	Ear Discharge	Hoarseness
History of Radiation	Ear infection	Sore Throat
Tension Headaches	Ruptured Ear Drum	Swelling in the Neck
Migraine Headaches	Decreased Hearing	Lymph Nodes Swollen
Hair Changes	Ringing in the Ears	Thyroid Problems
Glasses	Smell or Taste Change	Runny nose (except for colds)
Cataracts	Nasal Obstruction	
Glaucoma	Nasal polyps	
Night Sweats	Nose Bleeds	
Double Vision	Excessive Snoring	
Blurred Vision	Bleeding Gums	
Floaters/Black Spots in Eyes	Mouth Ulcers	

Cardiovascular System

Born With a Heart Problem	Waking Out of a Sound Sleep
Heart Murmur	Due to Shortness of Breath
Heart Valve Problem	Shortness of Breath When Lying
Rheumatic Fever What Age?	Flat
Inflammation of the Sac around	Swelling in the Ankles or Legs
the Heart or Heart Muscle	Fatigue Out of the Ordinary
Dizziness	Heart Attack – List Date(s)
Passing Out	Angioplasty (Balloon)/Stent -
Losing Consciousness	Date(s)
Known Heart Rhythms Problems	Bypass Surgery – List Date(s)
Palpitations, Skips, Flutters,	Chest Discomfort
Racing, Pounding	Aortic Aneurysm
Extreme Shortness of Breath on	Cerebral Aneurysm
Exertion	Abnormal Pulses
	in Your Arms or Legs
	Varicose Veins

Pulmonary System

Cough

Phlegm – What color?

Cough Up Blood

History of Radiation

Pain with Deep Breaths/Pleurisy

Wheezing

Asthma

Loud Noise with Breathing

Pneumonia

Bronchitis

TB or Positive TB Stan Test

COPD

Emphysema

Blood Clots in Lungs

Gastrointestinal System

Appetite – Good   Fair   Poor

Diet –   Good   Fair   Poor

Nausea/ Vomiting

Vomit Blood or Coffee Ground Material

Excessive Hiccups

Heart Burn or Indigestion

Trouble or Pain Swallowing/ Food Get Stuck in Your Threat

Hiatal Hernia

Abdominal Hernia

Belly Button Hernia

Esophageal Reflux

Esophageal Ulcer

Stomach Ulcer

Duodenal Ulcer

Jaundice

Hepatitis

Liver Disease

Gallbladder Disease

Pancreas Disease

Constipation (Other than occasional)

Diarrhea

Irritable Bowl Syndrome

Colitis or Crohn's Disease

Abdominal Pain

Rectal Pain

Black, Pasty Tarry Stools

Blood in Stools or in Toilet

Gas and/or Bloating

Hemorrhoids

Family history of Colon Cancer

Bowel Incontinence

Genitourinary System

Difficulty or Pain urinating	Lumps, Bumps or Tenderness
Burning when urinating	in the Testicles
Involuntary Delay or Inability	Penile Discharge
to Start Urinary Stream.	Pain on Erection
Have to Urinate Frequently	Peyronie's Disease
Urinate More Than 2 Times a	Impotence
Night	Ulcers
Have to Urinate Large	Menopause
Amounts Frequently	Menstrual Problems
Urinary Incontinence	Venereal Disease
Blood in the Urine	Kidney Stones – Side(s) L/R
Pus in the Urine	Flank Pain

Prostate Problems
Inguinal Hernia(s) - Side(s)
L/R
Breast Pain
Breast Discharge
Breast Mass
Breast Tenderness
Breast Dimpling
Lymph Nodes/Lumps in Arm
Pit
Enlarged Breast in Men

Muscles, Bones and Joints | Skin

Muscles, Bones and Joints		Skin
Osteoporosis (Decreased Bone)	Muscle Aches (Other than if you	Rash
Osteopenia (Decreased Calcium in	have over-used them)	Hives
the Bone)	Muscle Weakness	Moles
Disk Disease of the Spine	Muscle Swelling	Melanoma
Sciatica	Neck Pain	
Bursitis	Low Back Pain	Basal Cell Cancer
Scoliosis (Spine Curved to Left or	Bursitis	Squamous Cell Cancer
Right)		Eczema (Inflammation of the skin)
Kyphosis (Spine Curved Forward)		Acne
Lordosis (Hollow Back in Lumbar		Psoriasis
Region)		Contact Dermatitis
Joint Aches		Hair Changes
Hot, Red, Tender or Swollen Joints		Nail Fungus (Usually thick yellow
Gout		nails)
Osteoarthritis		Skin lumps or humps
Rheumatoid Arthritis		Lipoma (Fat Tumors)
Muscle Cramps		

Neurological

Seizure	Paralysis
Strokes	Tremors
TIAs	Seizure
Unsteady Gait	Strokes
Dizziness/Light headedness	TIAs
Vertigo	Unsteady Gait
Loss of Consciousness	Dizziness/Lightheadedness
Trouble Speaking	Vertigo
Disorientation	Loss of Consciousness
Hallucinations	Trouble Speaking
Memory Loss	Disorientation
Temporary Loss of Vision or	Hallucinations
Blindness	Memory Loss
Numbness or Tingling (Hands, Arms,	
Legs, Feet, etc.)	
Weakness of One or More Parts of	
the Body	

Blood Transfusions

Using your own blood

Other Notes: